Praise for the Alphabet Of Avoidance

"More like alphabet of common sense! And a quick read, too. No need to wade through depressing edicts or endless internet research when you have this no nonsense, fun, factually accurate riff on what most of us know we should do--for our health, our neighbor's health, and the health of our shared planet--but aren't yet doing. So jump in! Take it one letter at a time. Or race a friend to Z."

-**Alexandra Zissu**, *Author & Environmental Journalist*, www.alexandrazissu.com

"Lisa Borden is knowledgeable and passionate and her clever Alphabet spells out nothing less than a better quality of life. The most fun and useful pocket guide I've seen in a while!"

-**Rick Smith**, *Executive Director, Environmental Defence*, www.environmentaldefence.ca

"Lisa Borden is the voice of no-nonsense, common sense, low impact, conscious living. She makes it entertaining and easy. With every action suggested, Borden offers the best solution to make it happen. She is a resource of great brands, and the ultimate guru for how to make low-impact living incredibly time and cost effective. Michael Pollan penned the go-to guide for Food Rules, Borden is now offering us a go-to-guide for Intelligent Living. Her A-Z rules benefit both personal and environmental health and greatness. Reading the Alphabet of Avoidance will make us smart. Following it makes us brilliant."

-**Meghan Telpner**, *Nutritionista*, www.meghantelpner.com

"I think the Alphabet of Avoidance is a great idea and I hope people listen to it because it's worth listening to my mom. Trust me."

-**Ryan**, *age 11, Lisa Borden's son*

For Rob, Ryan, Joey and Andy,
who are my whole world,
inspire me every day to do better,
and continue to avoid
an increasingly long list of
everyday things by my side.

The Alphabet of Avoidance may be purchased for corporate, educational, or other promotional sales. For more information, contact Borden Communications www.bordencom.com

Concept + Text by Lisa Borden, Borden Communications + Design Inc.
Designed by Lisa Borden, Borden Communications + Design Inc.

TABLE OF CONTENTS

Once upon a time, necessity was the mother of invention. People lived a simple life, because life was simpler. Things were reusable because people cherished what they had, shopping was done locally because long distance travel wasn't an option, water was valued, and cleaning was done with lemons. Now, daily, at lightning speed, things become more complex - some change is positively incredible, but so much is scary. We live in an odd world. Most of us know that plastic bags, disposable water bottles, cleaning chemicals, and auto emissions are bad for our environment, and bad for us. Yet, we still drive cars, forget our reusable bags, buy water at the gym and spray toxic stuff onto our mirrors to try and clean them.

If you think about it, you'll realize that the world we live in is actually encouraging us to consume more in order to reduce our impact. Buy green. Try this. Throw this out. Never use that. Replace it now. Nope, that was wrong, now do this. Maybe you find it all stressful, maybe you find it overwhelming, but don't write off living healthier and smarter. It is absolutely worth buying into the green movement, and, it's just as important to know what to avoid.

Don't just blame the people who make this stuff. Blame the people who buy it. We control the way we shop and what we shop for and using our common sense will help us make more responsible purchases, or no purchases at all. Every dollar you spend is a vote for something...simple supply and demand. So, make sure to demand the right "goods" and avoid the wrong "stuff". **And, we all live happily ever after. The end.**

If you think you're too small to make a difference,
try sleeping in a room with a mosquito.
African Proverb

Do or not do, there is no try.
Yoda

We are what we repeatedly do.
Excellence, therefore, is not an act, but a habit.
Aristotle

Be who you are and say what you feel, because those
that matter don't mind, and those that mind don't matter.
Dr. Seuss

It's not that I'm so smart,
it's just that I stay with problems longer.
Albert Einstein

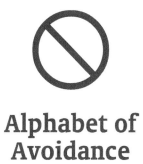

Alphabet of Avoidance

TAKE ACTION

**shop for safer personal care
products using this "wallet" sized guide**
http://bit.ly/nWacCU

**evaluate what you use, and
research safe alternatives**
www.ewg.org/skindeep

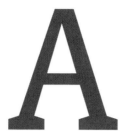

anti-perspirant

Do sweat the small stuff...that's how we can change the world. You may even perspire as you go through the pages of things to avoid! So, before you roll on, read the labels and ingredients on your deodorant (and all other personal care products). Do you know what they are? Can you pronounce everything? Are there parabens in there? Is there even a list? Remember, if it's on you, it's in you.

TAKE ACTION

find out *how* and *where* to recycle batteries
in your area, and why throwing them out
does more harm than good

http://earth911.com

B

batteries

Powering up all the gadgets in our lives with conventional batteries and then dumping them in landfills creates a toxic mess. Instead, try rechargeables, and take a look at wind powered, solar powered or hand crank eco-gadgets coming on the market with great force. If you do use batteries, make sure they are put in the right place when you are done with them.

TAKE ACTION

watch a great documentary that

will change your relationship with corn forever

www.kingcorn.net

read a little Marion Nestle,

it goes a long way

www.foodpolitics.com

C

---

corn

Go corn-free…we don't mean corn-on-the-cob, we mean corn-fed meat, corn-sweetened juice and pop, corn-oiled salad dressings, crackers and cereals with corn, corn syrups, corn solids, corn starches and more GMO, processed food product! Corn-stuff is in way too much of our food, especially from packages and restaurants, so this is a more challenging thing to steer clear of, but you won't believe how avoiding it will change your life (and our world).

TAKE ACTION

source the best tools

for eating on the go

http://bit.ly/pPfQW1

D

disposables

Buy cloth napkins to replace paper napkins. Buy a set of stainless steel chopsticks instead of wood ones in paper sleeves. Buy food safe and leakproof storage instead of using tin foil, plastic baggies and disposable containers. Ditch the plastic water bottles for a tried, tested and true refillable one. The choices are endless. You'll find reusables that suit your style and lifestyle...guaranteed.

TAKE ACTION

practice your kindness skills

www.boomboomcards.com

E

---

eco-bullying

Screaming with your arms flailing at an eco-sinner who is standing in the next aisle asking for their grocery items to be double plastic bagged makes you an eco-sinner, too. Rather than being angry and finger-wagging, promote eco-education with kindness and understanding. Awareness leads to more of us wanting and willing to do our part. Plus, charm always gets you further anyway.

TAKE ACTION

mist yourself, your stuff, and the air

with clean products like Graydon's Multi Mist

www.clinicalluxurybynature.com

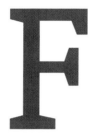

fragrance

If it stinks, it stinks. Perfumes and anything with the ingredient "fragrance" can contain parabens, phthalates and other synthetic compounds that experts label as harmful to our bodies (and our water when washed away). This includes body lotions, laundry products, and even some kids toys. As for air fresheners, don't mask odours with toxins - open the windows, that's as fresh as it gets!

TAKE ACTION

wrap up your presents in
lead-free, washable, fair-trade-made bags -
it's gorgeous gift wrap and a gift, all in one

www.rumebags.com

G

---

gift wrap

According to the Use Less Stuff Report, wrapping paper and shopping bags alone account for about 4 million tons of trash annually in the US. Even the production of it all causes harm - think of all of that ink and paper. Gift wrap is used for only such a brief time, and it's not even recyclable! Some may think reusing old gift wrap or giving an unwrapped gift is being lazy and cheap, but you can just use being "eco" as an excuse (to save money and our planet).

TAKE ACTION

find out where all your "stuff" comes from,

and where it goes afterwards

www.storyofstuff.com

watch how much you buy or you

may end up like these people

http://bit.ly/3Gt4c

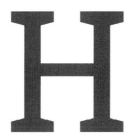

hoarding

We all have WAY too much stuff. If you have it and don't use it, donate it, swap it or sell it. If you don't have it and don't need it, don't buy it. Less stuff is good, good stuff is better, better stuff is enjoyable. Don't hoard...share or savour!

TAKE ACTION

support and protect your right

to breathe clean air

www.cleanair.org

develop an anti-idling campaign

at your school

http://bit.ly/pBWhET

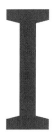

idling

Idling for more than 10 seconds burns gas twice as fast as driving for that same amount of time, and produces a great amount of toxic emissions into our air. So when you're stopped (think carpool, date drop-offs, take-out, pick-ups) it's usually worth turning off your engine. Idling gets us nowhere. Quickly.

TAKE ACTION

for the best kept secrets on

how to stop catalogues and all your junk

http://bit.ly/dfhCm2

J

junkmail

The name says it all..."junk"mail! Of course you need to get rid of it. The industry standard for a successful unaddressed advertising campaign is a 2% response rate, which means 98% of the resources making junk mail are wasted! You can put a stop to it right now - no cost to you, big savings for everyone.

TAKE ACTION

read more about why I think

single-use and single-purpose stuff sucks

http://bit.ly/efspoN

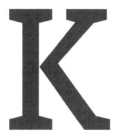

kitchen crap

You know the drawer in your kitchen filled with utensils that serve one single purpose and typically aggravate you more than serve you? If you want to cut the crusts off a sandwich, use a knife - you don't need a separate gadget to accomplish it, right?! If you simplify, it'll be easier to find everything you are looking for when you need it. Having the right tools means you won't need lots of little gimmicks.

TAKE ACTION

get yourself some BaaLLS

(and grab some for your friends, too!)

www.baalls.com

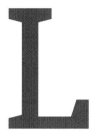

laundry dryer sheets

Fabric softeners, dryer sheets (and even dryer balls made from PVC) contain some not-so-snuggly ingredients. The warm fuzzy bunnies, teddy bears, or babies found on the front of packaging make us believe that they are safe and comforting, so we often overlook the fine print telling us that they contain hazardous chemicals. Make sure your fresh laundry is not in fact really dirty.

TAKE ACTION

protect your head from radiation,
while also protecting your phone. It's a win/win
www.pongcanada.com

find out where your electronics go
when you replace them
http://bit.ly/sUGKof

M

---

mobile phone mayhem

There are billions of us who are mobile phone subscribers and it increases every year. Children are starting to use technology and gadgets earlier and more frequently. It's alarming how dangerous the radiation from all of this is - and how many phones end up in landfill too quickly, just to keep up with the Joneses!

TAKE ACTION

if you need to paint your nails

try something water based

www.scotchnaturals.com and

www.hopscotchkids.com

N

nail polish

It's nice to feel pampered while at a spa, but brushing on a coat of formaldehyde, toluene and DBP (phthalate) nail polish is not something to feel relaxed about (maybe because it's strikingly similar to automotive paint!). Pick out polishes that are non-toxic and water based, or be the safest and skip painting your nails altogether. Watch out for removers too - what and how is it stripping?

TAKE ACTION

demand clean energy

http://bit.ly/qZWMt5

light clean candles

www.orbcandles.com

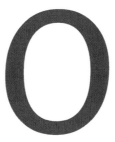

oil

Get off oil. We're not referring to cold-pressed, organic oils, we're talking about our dangerous addiction to oil - the kind that makes candles, petroleum jelly and plastics. Did you know that it takes 4 - 5 ounces of crude oil to produce one bottle that holds 18 ounces of water? (And even more oil is used to transport these bottles into stores and then home...gasp!). "O" also stands for Outrage, which you should feel considering crappy oil is in so much of our stuff, and really needs to get out.

TAKE ACTION

see it and believe it

http://bit.ly/MLtS

P

plastic produce bags

It's fantastic that you're bringing your own reusable bags for grocery shopping, but what about replacing those toxic throwaways for our produce and bulk? Don't suffocate your fresh produce! Our single-use plastics end up in floating bundles called "gyres" that not only clog our oceans, but get eaten by our fish, and our birds, and then up the food chain it goes! Not yum.

TAKE ACTION

spot the greenwashing sins
and become a smarter consumer
http://bit.ly/4legv5

Q

quasi-eco stuff

With too many "green", "eco", and "organic" products to even choose from, the best thing you can do for yourself is to learn to be an informed and active label reader. Understand and know what you are buying, where it came from and why you need it. If you can't understand any of that criteria, don't buy or buy into it. Common sense rules.

TAKE ACTION

calculate your water footprint

http://bit.ly/9tNZlH

R

running water

Turn the tap off while you brush your teeth...you don't flush the toilet the whole time you are sitting down, do you? Challenge yourself to a shorter shower, use less while washing dishes, and don't fill anything up higher than you need to, including your kettle.

TAKE ACTION

buy glass straws that come with

a lifetime guarantee ·

yes, they are that confident.

www.strawesome.com

S

straws

Yes, drinking straws can prevent lemon seeds from being swallowed (that's why they were invented), but do you really need that plastic thing in your drink and in your mouth? Plastic straws are really dangerous, too - there's a reason they aren't allowed at the zoo, you know. When your straw gets thrown away, where do you think "away" is?

TAKE ACTION

say no to unnecessary packaging and

fill your stomach, not our landfill

www.takeoutwithout.com

T

take-out

Take out the take out! Bring a litterless lunch from home, or enjoy dinner from your kitchen...just visualize all of the styrofoam, foil, cardboard, paper and plastic you'll avoid. If you are going to let a chef cook for you (we all like a break!), just take your own containers. Glass containers with lids rule. It's that easy and the best trend to hit the restaurant scene.

TAKE ACTION

lower your usage, meet your target,

and get rewarded for conserving

www.lowfoot.com

google "phantom energy" and

learn why it sucks (our power and in life)

U

utility charges

Unless you're living off the grid, utility charges are not completely avoidable, but when you see those office buildings all lit up at night, are there really that many people inside working? Be an influencer and get your workplace to turn off more. And, make sure you unplug as much as you can at home when not in use, even your cell phone charger sucks electricity when plugged in (whether you are charging it or not).

TAKE ACTION

**find out more on vocs and where
to find paint that doesn't stink
(plus over 400 other green actions)**

http://bit.ly/dJehnT

V

VOCS

VOCs are Volatile Organic Compounds. You can't see them, but they're all around us (sigh). They aren't listed as ingredients on our purchases and are most well-known for contributing to indoor pollution. Again, if it stinks, it stinks. Think new car smell, paint, toys, carpets, furnishings, vinyl shower curtains, and the list goes on and on. Evil.

TAKE ACTION

know what to look for on the label

http://bit.ly/pnuRtt

W

wearables

I'm not suggesting going commando, native, or stark naked, but making conventional fabrics can involve pesticides, formaldehyde, polyester, foams, dioxins and other yuckiness (wonder why some fibres can be so irritatingly uncomfortable?). The products we consume have an impact on our workers who make them, our communities, and our ecosystems, so know where your threads come from and what they are made of - quality, timeless fashion looks good and feels even better.

TAKE ACTION

read this greening-your-home-must-have

http://bit.ly/gwL42B

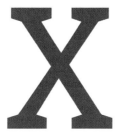

x-rated cleaners

Replace every conventional cleaner under the kitchen sink and in the laundry room with NOTHING (well, maybe not nothing, but as close to it as possible). There is a true, clear, easy and immediate fix – you can buy good, trustworthy brands of eco-friendly cleaners, or, it's even smarter to use microfibre cloths and water. If you are inclined, useingredients from your kitchen and make your own clean cleaning products. You do NOT have to sacrifice the cleanliness of your home.

TAKE ACTION

"like" the Healthwashing Wall of Shame -
post and expose your finds

http://on.fb.me/o5jful

Y

yucky fake food

If your grandmother wouldn't have immediately recognized it as "food" there's a good chance it's less food and more a manufactured "product". Who wants to eat a manufactured "good"? There's a reason that Cheez Whiz has a shelf life to rival the jar it's in! So, read labels and know what's in your food. Keep in mind that the items in the produce aisle don't have labels because they are as real as it gets.

TAKE ACTION

read why microwaved food is scary

http://scr.bi/ooD1BL

Z

zapping

It might be true that microwaves drain less energy than an oven, but it can't be good to nuke and zap your food, especially in plastic containers. Any packaged meal with microwave instructions is a sign to not eat it anyway. Heat up safely in ovens or on stoves - or eat something fresh like a salad!

FINAL WORDS

The beauty of life is that there are no final words. We can keep going, keep changing, keep learning, keep embracing the new, and of course, keep avoiding.

Any one change you make, or new service you try, is simply another beginning, not an ending point. And, when you like it and you feel that you've made a positive change, tell a few friends and all of a sudden, you will be making a big difference.

Start by supporting as many businesses (and people) that are local to you (and pleasant), who are making efforts to be green, and who provide quality products and services that aren't going to make us sick or contribute to an unhealthy planet.

Consider the following before you make purchases:

Country of Origin

How far did it travel to get onto the shelf? What are the working conditions like there? Are toxic chemicals like cadmium found in products from that country?

Labeling

As a general rule, if you can't pronounce the ingredient, you shouldn't be using it. If there is not a complete list, this is a strong indication that it is not a responsible purchase. Beware of claims such as "natural", "biodegradable" and even "organic", plus all of those eco-certifications as they unfortunately don't mean as much as a clear ingredient list that makes sense to you.

Packaging

Is the food in a glass or plastic jar? Are you paying for packaging or what's actually inside? Hint: pudding cups with pictures of animated characters on it are probably not going to be better for our health and our planet's happiness than a homemade one with fresh ingredients!

Other Options

Is there an organic or less packaged, less processed version close by? Compare labels. Don't get caught in the debate that surrounds us daily about the health impacts of our purchases, just choose to simplify. *The Precautionary Principle* teaches us that if we wait until we're absolutely certain something is not acceptable, we've probably waited too long.

Research and Perspective

Use QR codes and safe shopping apps to learn more about what you are buying, and visit sites like EWG's Cosmetics Database to learn about what's in your personal care products. Watch Story of Stuff and share it with friends and family. Ask questions about what you are buying, and demand answers.

Instead of depending on large corporations or experts to tell us that we need, rely on yourself - you are your own best expert (possibly hypocritical as I'm telling you what to do?). Just a reminder: We control the way we shop, and what we shop for and using our common sense will help us make more responsible purchases that will in turn save us time, save us money, save our health, and positively impact our shared world. How is that for good sense?

INDEX

AVOIDANCE ACCOMPLISHMENTS

Use this as a to-do list, or as a journal of the things you are avoiding!

ACKNOWLEDGEMENTS

Writing is a challenge for me. Not just because I have no formal training, or because I didn't do well in school, but because I have so much to say, and so little time to get it down on paper simply and clearly.

I must first and foremost thank my wonderful associate Alex Green, who kindly and professionally went through every draft of this book with me. She not only read over and edited the written words, but acted as my sounding board, listening to my thoughts and ideas (sometimes barely coherent ones) and made insightful suggestions for many letters of "my" Alphabet.

Special thanks also goes to all of my friends, family, clients, colleagues and online community who give me the non-stop inspiration to write, tweet and rant. Your names are too many to list here, but if you have listened to me (with or without rolling your eyes), supported me, hired me, retweeted me, commiserated with me, laughed with me or have given me a hug, I am always here to do the same for you.

And lastly, to the four most important people in my world, Rob, Ryan, Joey and Andy, who make everything possible - all I do is for you.